Dry Eye Relief

Dr. Glen Swartwout

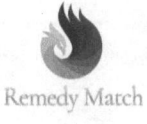

Remedy Match

Healing Oasis

Book Cover by Dr. Glen Swartwout

4th edition 2024

Also by

The Five Elements of Spiritual Development
The Hard Question of Consciousness
The Arrow of Time

Table of Contents

Preface

This book began as research notes for a presentation to the International College of Applied Nutrition in Tokyo, Japan, while I was establishing the Optometric Center of Tokyo to bring my father's pioneering work in natural eye and vision care to the Orient.

The book took further form through many years of clinical practice of Holistic Optometry and European Biological Medicine, as well as while co-authoring Natural Eye Care: An Encyclopedia, with Dr. Marc Grossman, O.D., L.Ac.

The Results:

After experiencing an Accelerated Self Healing™ program, author Joy Gardner wrote:

"You really helped me when I had the supposedly incurable Sjogren's Syndrome."

Joy is the author of the popular book, <u>The New Healing Yourself: Natural Remedies for Adults and Children</u>.

She is also known for her book <u>Vibrational Healing Through the Chakras</u>

Introduction

The purpose of this book is to provide an overview of insights and resources for potential therapies in the healing of the underlying causes of dry eye syndrome in all its many variations, which are ultimately unique to each person, and to some degree changing in time through the course of the condition and its healing. This is especially true in accelerated self-healing, where causal stress patterns are identified individually in real time, and the body's healing processes are supported with natural remedies like those introduced in this book based on functional response testing which is ultimately a form of biocommunication.

Remedies found to be effective in an individual case will never be limited to those identified in this book, since the causal chains present in the whole person must be treated, not just a presenting or salient symptom, which may well be at the effect or 'tail end' of causality.

Nevertheless, for both the clinician and the patient seeking palliative relief of symptoms or remedy possibilities particular to an individual or challenging case, this book is intended to offer an array of options to test and consider. In particular, the natural remedies in this book can readily be applied with adherence to the primary dictum of healing, "Primum non nocere."

Dedication

This book is dedicated to my Apprentice and Partner, Rae Luscombe, who has known the challenges of Dry Eye since suffering from Bell's Palsy when she literally froze her face in the cold North country of Canada from where she hails. She will be a ray of light, help, and hope for you as she has been in my life for over a quarter of a century. Our mission together is to end blindness and other suffering by healing the root causes.

Chapter 1

Solutions

Research shows that unpreserved eye drops enhance corneal healing and improve dry eye problems in comparison to preserved products. Fortunately, several unpreserved tear substitutes are available, including VIVA drops (which contain 19 I.U. of vitamin A per drop) and several single-dose tubes. Concern has been expressed, however, about the risk of corneal abrasion by the sharp ends of single-dose tubes. Among the other problems with eye drops is that 80% of people have difficulty getting them in the eyes, and even with practice 49% continue to have poor aim. Less than a third have even been shown how to do it right! The best method is to pull down the lower lid so the drop can be instilled onto the lower cul de sac (blind pouch) of the conjunctiva rather than directly onto the cornea. For those who have difficulty, eye drop guides are available to assist. For those who are unable to open their eyes while drops are instilled, drop them into the inner corner of the closed lids, and the drops will enter the eyes upon opening. Keep drops refrigerated if you experience stinging on instillation. Be sure to keep your eye drops separate from any similar-looking bottles, and to prevent contamination, be very careful not to touch the dropper with anything, including fingers or the eye itself. Look for a ring of dirt between the cap and lid as a sign that contamination has probably occurred. Be sure to wash your hands before using eye drops and keep the bottle in a clean place.

Nearly one out of three bottles become contaminated and should be replaced with a clean, fresh supply.

Blinking and tearing following the use of an eye drop can dilute the remedy to less than 1% of its original concentration in just a few minutes. To optimize therapeutic effectiveness after instillation, don't blink, but rather close the eyes for up to 2 minutes. You can even pinch gently at the root of the nose to prevent drainage through the tear ducts, increasing effectiveness by 65%. This is also a perfect time to help the eyes relax and improve circulation to the eyes with techniques like palming, eye stretch, and acupressure or shiatsu eye massage. Between applications, it is important to blink frequently and fully, as this spreads the tears over the front of the eye, moistening any dry areas. The normal tear break-up time (BUT) is over 10 seconds, permitting that length of staring before the cornea begins to show dry spots. With dry eye syndrome, this often shortens to just a few seconds. Staring also contributes to visual stress and is related to increases in myopia.

Related eye muscle tension may further reduce circulation in the eye area. There are three common hypotheses for the cause of dry eye:

Dry spots on the ocular surface; Inflammation of the eye surface;

Elevated tear film osmolarity (salinity) with loss of water from the tear film

Dry spots are associated with but don't cause dry eye, as half of dry eye patients have enough tear film stability to prevent dry spots between blinks.

Lemp MA, Hamill JR: Factors affecting tear film breakup in normal eyes. Arch Ophthalmol 89:103-105, 1973.

Dry eye surface disease is most severe within the palpebral aperture, but there are also changes on the superior and inferior bulbar conjunctiva, where dry spots do not occur. Rabbit studies show that loss of the corneal cell surface proteins that make the cornea wettable is a late change in dry eye disease.

In the 1800s, Hass theorized that dry eye was caused by a direct immune or inflammatory assault on the eye surface and that the changes on the eye surface are unrelated to the decrease in tear production. This hypothesis was intriguing until researchers started looking at ocular surface pathology in dry eyes. Surface pathology in patients who develop dry eye after having their lacrimal glands removed for epiphora (which is why this

operation went out of favor) and in patients with Sjogren's syndrome. The group with iatrogenic disease had exactly the same ocular surface changes as the Sjögren's group.

Scherz W, Dohlman CH: Is the lacrimal gland dispensable? Keratoconjunctivitis sicca after lacrimal gland removal. Arch Opthalmol 93:281-283, 1975.

In rabbits, every ocular surface change in Sjögren's syndrome is manifest in normal rabbits by raising tear film osmolarity, whether by blocking tear secretion, decreasing corneal sensation, or inducing meibomian gland dysfunction. Research shows an expression of inflammatory mediators (cytokines) on the eye surface in dry eyes, but inflammation is a non-specific response to any tissue damage. Inflammation helps clean up the damage. Increases in tear film osmolarity cause the increase of pro-inflammatory cytokines on the eye surface. There is no primary immune-inflammatory attack on the eye surface in dry eyes.

Dursun D, Wang M, Monroy D, Li D, Lokeshwar BL, Stern M, Pflugfelder SC: Experimentally induced dry eye produces ocular surface inflammation and epithelial disease. Adv Exp Med Biol 506(PtA):647-55, 2002.

When Sjögren first described the ocular surface pathology in dry eye, he concluded that it looked as if some "force" was pulling water across the ocular surface epithelium. It turns out that force was the osmotic force created by the osmotic gradient created by an elevation of tear film osmolarity. The ocular surface disease in dry eye is dependent on and proportional to elevations in tear film osmolarity.

Elevated tear film osmolarity causes the ocular surface changes in dry eyes. Farris finds that tear film osmolarity in dry eye patients increases through the course of each day.

Farris RL, Stuchell RN, Mandel ID. Tear osmolarity variation in the dry eye. Trans Am Ophthalmol Soc (United States) 84: p250-68, 1986.

The Tear Film

There are three layers to the normal tear film that keep the front surface of the eye comfortably lubricated and optically clear. The first is a lipid (oil) layer which prevents

tears from evaporating. This is secreted by the meibomian glands. The middle and thickest layer is the aqueous or watery layer, secreted by the lachrymal gland. The third layer, which binds the tears to the surface of the eye by making the eye tissue wettable, is a protein layer called mucin. This is secreted directly from the conjunctival surface on the white of the eye by goblet cells.

Dry eye syndrome is often related to other health conditions in the body. It is commonly associated with dryness of other mucus membranes (see Sjogren's syndrome, below) and even interior body surfaces like joints (arthritis). Many dry eye patients also complain of connective tissue problems like brittle nails and many experience skin sensitivity to detergents. Digestive imbalances and autoimmune processes like Sjogren's syndrome and lupus are frequently discovered underlying dry eye symptoms. When dry eye symptoms improve, there is also frequently noted an improvement in sinus and post-nasal drip conditions.

Sjogren's syndrome is considered the most commonly misdiagnosed of all health conditions in women over the age of 40, affecting 4 million Americans. In Sjogren's syndrome, dry eye symptoms are accompanied by dryness in other parts of the body. This cluster of symptoms is produced by an autoimmune process in which antibodies attack fluid-secreting cells. These glandular cells can ultimately be destroyed, and occasionally even become cancerous. A dry eye may be accompanied by fatigue, dry mouth (perhaps with a sore throat and swelling of the parotid gland), dry joints (arthritis), dry skin, dry, cracked lips, dry scalp (dandruff), and dry, brittle nails. Lack of saliva can lead to dental carries. Doctors may prescribe anti-inflammatory and immunosuppressive steroids. In advanced cases, cyclosporin may be prescribed as well. Allergy to drugs, especially penicillin, may be linked to Sjogren's syndrome.

Chapter 2

Limits of Conventional Care

Dry eye syndrome is one of the most common eye conditions. In 1990, about 33 million Americans experienced varying degrees of dry eye symptoms. By 1997 that figure increased to an alarming 59 million. The symptoms may include dryness, grittiness, irritation, burning, and even excessive tearing or watering. While many people find temporary relief with artificial tear preparations, this only palliates the symptoms, and preservatives found in many of these products can even aggravate the condition itself. In fact, these preservatives can kill corneal cells. Recovery of corneal health after exposure to preservatives takes a full week, while the conjunctiva takes up to 2 months to heal. The common eye drop preservative benzalkonium chloride causes worsening of dry eyes, making one more and more dependent on the use of such drops. This preservative, along with thimerosal and Tween, occurs in toxic concentrations in eye drops. Other pharmaceutical ingredients in eye drops contribute to dry eyes, too. Vasoconstrictors that 'get the red out' reduce circulation in the eye, decrease the production of the tear film, and worsen dry eye symptoms.

Many doctors recommend treatments that can include placing silicone plugs to block the eyes' tear ducts and even cauterizing the ducts closed to retain moisture in the eye. While such treatments do reduce the amount of artificial tears needed for many with severely dry eyes, it may merely mean applying drops every 4 hours or more rather than every 3 hours or less. Humidifiers may be helpful in dry or air-conditioned environments, and special moisture chamber goggles can also be worn to minimize tear evaporation. Even neutral gray wrap-around sun goggles may offer some relief, especially from aggravation by sun, wind, and dust. Side shields reduce evaporation by up to 40%. Perhaps if we look a little deeper at the pathophysiology and biochemistry of tears and tear production, we will find healthier solutions for many dry eye sufferers.

Chapter 3

Risk Factors

The aging process, which involves free radical damage to body tissues, increases the prevalence of dry eye symptoms. As we get older, on average our eyes produce 40% less lubrication. Pregnancy can also trigger dry eyes. Environmental allergens, toxins, and other irritants, like exposure to air conditioning, wind, excessive sunlight, dust, contact lenses, dry airplane air, smog and smoke contribute as well. Residents of the most polluted cities have increased risk of dry eye.

In one study 40% of dry eye patients were smokers. Second hand cigarette smoke also reduces the breakup time of the tears by 40%. Even a single cigarette can produce a level of carbon monoxide of 400 ppm (parts per million). Carbon monoxide, along with smog and chemical fumes inactivate lysozyme, the natural antibiotic secreted in the tears. Eye makeup, typically made of synthetic chemicals, depletes the lipid layer of the tears. Eye makeup is also frequently contaminated with bacteria.

Many synthetic medications also trigger dry eye. These include oral contraceptives and other estrogens, sympathomimetic agents, anticholinergic drugs like atropine and scopolamine, synthetic vitamin

A analogs (isotretinoin or Acutane), diuretics (especially those that deplete potassium), codeine, morphine, antihistamines, deconges-tants (including eye drops like visine, murine, prefrin and clear eyes), marijuana, cancer drugs and radiation treatments, phenothiazines, tranquilizers and antidepressants (like valium and elavil), glaucoma medications (including timoptic or timolol, betoptic, betagan and ocupress) and other beta blockers like practolol.

Pesticides and other petrochemical xeno-estrogens may also be a problem, so avoidance of commercial produce is recommended as much as possible. When organic produce is unavailable, peeling grapes and strawberries in particular is recommended due to the common use of persistent fungicides such as captan.

Mechanical problems with the eyelids such as scars, drooping lids (sometimes even due to pressure from eyeglass nosepads), sleeping with the eyelids partially open, and incomplete closure on blink can cause dry eyes. Neurological problems like Bell's palsy (paralysis of the facial nerve) can interfere with lid function, too.

Chapter 4

Lifestyle, Stress Management & Exercise

Ergonomic factors like the height of computer screens can affect dry eye symptoms, due to effects on eyelid positioning and resultant tear evaporation. Computers also double visual stress compared to conventional deskwork, which can involve increased staring. When reading or looking at a digital screen, the blink rate goes down to about 4 times a minute from 16 times.

Functional visual stress including focusing issues and problems with binocular eye teaming can also contribute to dry eye symptoms, as documented in a study by Hom and Lowell on patients with Acquired Brain Injury and Binocular Dysfunction. Severe dry eye symptoms were measured with a validated questionnaire: the Ocular Surface Disease Index, or OSDI.

Behavioral and Developmental Optometrists who practice Vision Therapy will be best able to help with both diagnosis and remediation of this important aspect of dry eye syndrome. The College of Optometrists in Vision Development and the Optometric Extension Program Foundation are good organizations to contact if you need referral to a local practitioner.

Electromagnetic fields from computers contribute to the overall stress pattern, and the resulting stress can be alleviated with a variety of technologies including ultra-low radiation computer monitors and even special computer software. For more on the issues and solutions with electromagnetic fields, see my book Electromagnetic Pollution Solutions.

Even vitamin A, important for mucin production, is used up more rapidly in the eye during computer work due to the invisible flickering of the screen. A number of nutritional factors play a role and will be discussed next.

Chapter 5

Milieu: Water & Biological Terrain

Symptoms of dryness generally tend to be associated with an overly alkaline state in the body tissues. Since active metabolism produces acidity in the form of Carbonic Acid (carbon dioxide dissolved in water), excess alkalinity is typically an indicator of blocked cellular respiration, most often due to blockade of the mitochondrial electron transport chain by a key toxin such as a heavy metal. Mercury is a common one seen clinically since it is the most symptomatic of toxins in the mineral kingdom and commonly encountered from environmental, dietary, and iatrogenic sources. Mercury is very often associated with Sjogren's Syndrome, which often expresses dryness not only in the eyes but also in the oral cavity and vaginal area.

Irritation, a common symptom that accompanies dry eyes can also be associated with a hyperacidic pH. While at first glance, this appears contradictory to the association of alkalinity with dryness, the meta-view sees both of these states as dynamic stages in pH dysregulation which is seen in states of toxicity (acidity) leading to deeper pathology (alkalinity). For vision therapists, it is the equivalent of the eso-exo swing sometimes seen in the course of treating strabismus and other binocular dysfunctions.

When testing electrophysiological measures on the acupuncture meridians, we see this same classical pattern on occasion, even in the balancing of a disordered impedance value with a series of causal remedies. A low impedance value, described in German Diagnostic Electroacupuncture as an indicator of a degenerative state, may progress through a hyper impedance value (inflamed) before it settles into the clinically normal, sustainable range.

Symptomatically, this also corresponds to the cleansing reaction or healing crisis, and what we call Negative Regulation in European Biological Medicine.

See detailed discussion of the 5 Phases of Health and Disease in my DVDs and other books for important background on the terrain as expressed in the proton, electron, and photon content of the body's water. Even simple dehydration, contributed to by intake of alcohol, sugar, caffeine, and soda, contributes to Dry Eye Syndrome. On the therapeutic side, intake of rejuvenating alkaline, anti-oxidant, micro-structured water helps to restore tissue hydration.

Chapter 6

Diet, Food Sensitivities and Allergies

Digestion

Digestive function is impaired in Sjogren's syndrome patients, including deficiencies in hydrochloric acid and pepsin. Resultant hypochlorhydria symptoms include bloating, gas, and nausea, as well as allergies and depression associated with Sjogren's syndrome.

Herbal bitters and homeopathic remedies like Digestzymes help stimulate the secretion of digestive juices. Digestive enzyme supplementation (substitution therapy) has even been suggested except when stomach ulcers or pain are present. In some cases, the underlying cause may be a bacterial parasite in the stomach, called helicobacter pylori. Correction of such an infestation may involve anti-parasitic remedies, like Artemisia & Clove, or antibiotics along with steps to correct the terrain, so that it is not so susceptible to reinfestation.

Acidophilus, bifidus, and other friendly bacterial flora supplements are recommended in general to improve the function and terrain of the gastrointestinal tract. Three capsules a day of Friendly Flora are recommended.

Sugar & Artificial Sweeteners

Sugar (sucrose) intake increases the risk of dry eye by decreasing the tear break-up time, especially when the diet also includes less folic acid. Consumption of more than 11 teaspoons/day of sucrose (most of which is hidden in prepared foods) is the second most significant factor (after folic acid) linked to reduced tissue potassium levels in dry eye patients (see mineral section). Note that a single can of soda contains about 9 teaspoons of sugar! Thus avoidance of sweet processed foods while eating more leafy green vegetables can help improve dry eyes.

Avoidance of aspartame (Nutrasweet) also improves dry eye symptoms and contact lens tolerance in many patients. This can also alleviate a commonly associated symptom of intense thirst. Is it possible that aspartame makes diet soda addictive due to this side- effect of thirst? This may boost sales, but the FDA receives more letters complaining of side effects from aspartame than any other drug on the market!

Photosensitizing Foods

Certain foods may also exacerbate light sensitivity in Sjogren's syndrome patients. These particular foods, including limes, celery, and parsley, contain furocoumarins, which are natural compounds that can increase photosensitivity.

Diet

In one study, only 18% of dry eye patients ate leafy green vegetables and only 6% ate fruits. At the same time, 75% were exposed to direct sunlight for over six hours a day. In addition, 72% were strictly vegetarian, lacking a full complement of essential amino acids as well as certain beneficial oils in their diet. These essential nutrients are crucial to the proper function of the mucin and lipid layers of the tear film. In general, a broad spectrum, optimum potency nutritional supplement should be taken as the basis of building an effective supplementation program.

Chapter 7

Neuroprotection

The extreme discomfort of Dry Eyes is largely attributable to the fact that the cornea hosts more nerve endings per square millimeter than any other part of the body. Since neuroprotection is an essential element of healing treatments for dry eye, one of the beauties of natural medicine is that most nutrients, homeopathic remedies and botanicals have more side benefits than undesirable side effects. Thus, for example, the Omega 3 fatty acids that help reduce inflammation also help with the oil layer of the tears and are the dominant fatty acids in healthy nerve cells.

When the sensory nerves of the cornea, a branch of the Trigeminal Nerve (cranial nerve V) are damaged by Dry Eye Syndrome, this can result in reduced reflex tear production by the lacrimal gland. This can be a factor in diabetes, viral infections of the cornea and other underlying causal processes.

For peripheral neuropathy issues like this, we formulated Nerve Pulse.

Chapter 8

Free Electrons &
Antioxidants

Antioxidant enzyme levels are low in the conjunctival cells in Dry Eye Syndrome. Supplementation

Tear stability and ocular surface status improved with oral antioxidant supplementation (P<0.05). Absolute increase in tear stability correlated with absolute change in goblet cell density. Symptoms were improved by placebo, but objective findings were not affected. (Blades KJ, Patel S, Aidoo KE. Oral antioxidant therapy for marginal dry eye. Eur J Clin Nutr. 2001 Jul;55(7):589-97.)

One specific anti-oxidant recommendation is Astaxanthin 6 mg daily for more advanced dry eye as well as dry eye related to prolonged close work.

We include Astaxanthin in our Macular Wellness product series, each of which supplies a single carotenoid to ensure that they don't compete for absorption.

Our Vitamin C Syntropy formula is actually a complete intracellular antioxidant formulation.

We also strongly recommend upgrading your water to alkaline ionized water that is high in Molecular Hydrogen, which is the ultimate and perfect antioxidant. You can learn more at RemedyMatch.com.

Chapter 9

Reverse AGEing: Antiglycation

Sugar regulation is a major factor in Dry Eye Syndrome, including a high incidence in diabetes. Therapy involves avoidance of refined sugars and artificial sweeteners, correction of sugar metabolism at the cellular and regulatory levels, as well as protection against glycation which is a degenerative change in the connective tissues with the formation of AGE (Advanced Glycation Endproducts). One can of soda contains about 9 teaspoons of sugar. Caffeine and chocolate, even if they are not taken with added sugar, which is rare, have an even stronger effect on the sugar regulating response of the pancreas than pure sugar itself, so I also recommend avoiding these and any other stimulants.

Our dynamic duo for this major root cause of so many issues including dry eyes, is Glucose Tolerance and Reverse AGE.

Chapter 10

Immune Modulators

Inflammation of both the glands and the ocular surface is a major factor in Dry Eye Syndrome. Autoimmunity in Dry Eye is linked to resistance of Th17 T-cells to regulatory T-cells. This produces elevated inflammatory interleukin-17+. IL-17 is also linked to rheumatoid arthritis and multiple sclerosis.

Immune modulators normalize the immune function by reducing hyperresponses such as inflammation, autoimmune processes, and allergy while increasing the effectiveness of immunity against pathogens. See Materia Medica for more specifics on immune modulators like phytosterols that are removed from virtually all commercial oils in the modern diet.

Check out the dozens of immune modulators included in our Immune Modulation formula!

Chapter 11

Minerals

Hypochlorhydria, linked to Sjogren's syndrome, reduces the ability to absorb many minerals including calcium, magnesium and zinc. In 1983, Graeme Wilson and his associates found that the minerals calcium, magnesium, potassium and sodium were each essential and together provide sufficient mineral content in the tear film to promote integrity of the corneal epithelium.

Calcium

Calcium stores are depleted by eating refined sugar, as well as excess sodium from junk foods. Magnesium is also essential in regulating calcium metabolism, as is modest exposure to ultraviolet light as in full spectrum lighting, or a 15 minute daily walk.

Calcium is needed to maintain strong connective tissues, such as the cornea and conjunctiva, as well as for sugar regulation, balancing of pH, and proper nerve and muscle function. It is also present in the tear film itself.

Chromium

Glucose-tolerance-factor (GTF) chromium is critical for metabolism and regulation of sugars, yet it is one of the first nutrients lost in the refining of foods such as grains.

Refined sugar also increases the loss of chromium in the urine, leading to increased risks for reduced life span, cardiovascular disease and diabetes.

Magnesium

Magnesium is required for regulation of intracellular potassium supplies, for sugar metabolism, for the activation of vitamin B6 into its active form, pyridoxal-5-phosphate (P5P), and for the production of prostaglandin E-1. The most absorbable form of magnesium supplement is magnesium glycinate.

Potassium

Potassium is a critical intracellular mineral, needed for many functions including sugar metabolism and maintenance of the cell's electrical membrane potential. Potassium levels measured in hair tissue average 9 ppm for dry eye patients compared to a level of 65 ppm average for controls. This is linked to low intake of folic acid, ascorbic acid and vitamin B6, along with high sugar consumption. If dietary potassium intake is less than 4,000 mg/day, it is recommended to increase consumption of fresh fruit and vegetables. One banana contains about 400 mg of potassium, and all fruits and vegetables are high in this important mineral.

Conventional diuretic medications as well as aspirin deplete potassium. Supplementation with vitamin C and vitamin B6 can produce diuresis when desired clinically, while improving dry eye. Sodium Sodium is a major constituent of the aqueous layer of the tear film.

Zinc

Zinc and Vitamin A are synergistic. An animal study assesses the interaction between zinc and vitamin A on the ocular surface:

Zinc, Vitamin A and the Ocular Surface Group Diet Microscopy

    1. vitamin A and zinc normal

    2. zinc decrease epithelial microvilli; corneal keratinization

    3. zinc decrease epithelial microvilli

    4. vitamin A decrease epithelial microvilli

    5. vitamin A decrease epithelial microvilli

(Kanazawa S, Kitaoka T, Ueda Y, et. al. Interaction of zinc and vitamin A on the ocular surface. Graefes Arch Clin Exp Ophthalmol 2002;240(12):1011-21)

We include both Vitamin A and Zinc in all of our eye drop formulations, along with other synergistic ingredients.

Chapter 12

Vitamins

A

Vitamin A is normally found in the tear film. In parts of the world where vitamin A deficiency is widespread, severe dry eye syndrome is a leading cause of blindness. Vitamin A is needed for the health of all epithelial (surface) tissues, as well as for good night vision. Sjogren's syndrome is often associated with decreased night vision performance, and this may be due to low levels of vitamin A and B vitamins as well, resulting from liver dysfunction. Vitamin A is especially needed to produce the mucin layer of the tears. Beta carotene (pro-vitamin A) has been reported to be helpful in dry eye as well. Eye drops containing vitamin A, together with vitamin C, have also been reported to improve dry eye syndrome. Vitamin A metabolism is dependent on Zinc.

B complex

B vitamin deficiency is linked to Sjogren's syndrome due to associated liver dysfunction. B1

Vitamin B1 (thiamine) is needed for the metabolism of sugars but is deficient in refined foods loaded with refined sugar. Whole foods that contain high sugar levels, such as sweet fruits, also contain the needed vitamin B1 for the body to metabolize those sugars without depleting the vitamin in the process.

B2

Supplemental vitamin B2 has been recommended. B3

Vitamin B3 (niacin) taken in excess can exacerbate dry eye symptoms. It is generally best to take any B vitamins with a full B complex supplement so that deficiencies of other B vitamins are not induced.

B6

Vitamin B6 (pyridoxine) is needed for the proper absorption of magnesium, which is required in the maintenance of potassium levels in the cells. Both vitamin B6 and magnesium are needed in the body's production of prostaglandin E-1. B6 is also required for sugar metabolism, so refined foods containing sugar deplete this vitamin. Dietary intake of less than 2 mg/day of vitamin B6 is the fourth most significant food factor linked to low potassium in dry eyes (see mineral section). If dietary intake is less than 4 mg/day, increasing high protein foods rich in vitamin B6 are suggested, including raw walnuts, hazelnuts, spinach, or rare grass-fed beef steak. Medium to well-done proteins result in increased demand for vitamin B6. In 1978, Ned Paige first reported improvement of dry eye syndrome with high doses of vitamin B6 in many patients.

Vitamin B6, together with vitamin C and essential fatty acids, has been found to improve dry eye symptoms and tear production. In one study, tear production almost doubled in the first month among dry eye patients taking up to 50 mg/day of vitamin B6 together with EPO and vitamin C.

B12

Vitamin B12 deficiency caused by malabsorption associated with digestive dysfunction in Sjogren's syndrome may help to explain the associated fatigue and depression symptoms. A dosage of 1,000 to 1,500 mcg/day is recommended.

Folic Acid

Folic acid is needed for cell mitosis (reproduction, such as for tissue repair) as well as sugar metabolism. Dietary intake of less than 310 mcg/day of food folate is the number

one food factor associated with reduced potassium levels (see mineral section). If intake is less than 500 mcg/day, it is recommended to increase consumption of raw fresh fruits and vegetables. Leafy greens, sprouts, and raw fruit are especially high in this commonly deficient and heat-sensitive vitamin.

C

Vitamin C is concentrated in the tear film to a higher level than that found in the blood. It protects the eye from oxidative stresses, including toxins, irritants, allergens, and inflammation. Vitamin C is a necessary cofactor for the final phase of production of prostaglandin E-1. Vitamin C is also needed for proper sugar metabolism.

Hypochlorhydria, linked to Sjogren's syndrome, reduces absorption of vitamin C. In one study, exposure to ammonia fumes reduced the vitamin C concentration in the tears by 50%. Dietary intake of vitamin C below 175 mg/day is the third greatest food factor (after folic acid deficiency and sugar toxicity) linked to reduced potassium levels in dry eye patients. Increased vitamin C intake is definitely suggested if the diet contains less than 400 mg/day. Dr. Ben C. Lane recommends eating more raw, fresh fruits and vegetables. Oral supplementation at optimum levels helps the eye heal its surface and connective tissues. For example, one study found that while 50 mg/day had no effect, 1500 mg/day greatly increased the healing of corneal ulcerations. Vitamin C, together with vitamin B6 and essential fatty acids, has been found to improve dry eye symptoms and tear production. In one study, tear production almost doubled in the first month among dry eye patients taking up to 7,500 mg/day of vitamin C together with EPO and vitamin B6. Eye drops containing vitamin C together with vitamin A have also been reported to improve dry eye syndrome.

E

Absorption of vitamin E may be reduced by deficient secretion of pancreatin and bile. Oil-based vitamin E supplements can go rancid if not refrigerated, counteracting the desired effects of the vitamin. Dry vitamin E (succinate form) is also more easily absorbed and utilized. Natural vitamin E (d form) is preferred over synthetic (dl) because half of the synthetic vitamin E molecules have the opposite shape of normal vitamin E, reducing effectiveness, and perhaps producing other forms of metabolic or energetic interference in the body. Topical vitamin E has been recommended for dry skin in Sjogren's syndrome and has been used successfully in combination with other nutrients in eye drop form for dry eye patients.

Chapter 13

Essential Fatty Acids

Essential fatty acids are needed to produce both the lipid layer and the aqueous layer of the tear film. The omega-6 fatty acid gamma linolenic acid (GLA), found in evening primrose oil and human breast milk, is also a precursor for the prostaglandin PGE-1.

Deficiency of pancreatin and bile secretion reduces absorption of these essential nutrients, as well as vitamin E, from the diet.

Studies have found that about half or more of all dry eye sufferers achieve improvement in symptoms like reduced tear production, dry eye, visual acuity, brittle nails and skin sensitivity to detergents as early as 10 days after beginning supplementation with omega- 6 essential fatty acids from evening primrose oil (EPO) together with vitamin C and vitamin B6.

In another study, tear production almost doubled in the first month among dry eye patients taking 3,000 mg/day of EPO together with vitamin C and vitamin B6. Symptoms tend to relapse eventually among patients who discontinue supplementation. Eating more small, cold water fish, flax seeds and walnuts, as well as supplementation with products like EPA fish oil, flax seed oil, borage oil and EPO is recommended.

Omega-3's produce an increase in tear break-up time (TBUT), which is the amount of time it takes for dry spots to appear on the eye after a person blinks. At 30 days, TBUT increased from a mean of 3.9 seconds to 5.7 seconds with supplementation, versus 4.5 to 4.7 in the control group. This is 71% improvement for patients taking omega-3s versus 3.3% without (p<0.001).

Scores on the Ocular Surface Disease Index (OSDI), which measures dry eye symptoms and disability due to these symptoms, improved by 26% with Omega-3 treatment, and worsened by 4% in the control group (p=0.004). Schirmer's score, a measure of eye surface wetness, improved by 22.3% in the Omega-3 group and 5.1% in the placebo group (p=0.033).

One author suggests a dosage of 500 to 1000 mg/day of fish oil, EPO or flax seed oil for those with Sjogren's syndrome. Another recommends 6 capsules a day of EPO in divided doses for between 1 and 12 weeks if needed in addition to increased intake of organic raw, fresh foods. Another suggested target is 1500 to 1800 mg EPA/DHA in Triglyceride form to bring the Omega index over 9%.

Oxidized, rancid, and toxic fats from commercial red meat and dairy products, fried foods, and hydrogenated oils like margarine compete and interfere with the proper function of the essential fatty acids. They should be eliminated from the diet as much as possible.

My favorite EFA remedy is our WholOmega which supplies Omega 3 as DHA from algae. DHA is the main fatty acid needed in the eyes and the brain. Because algae are at the base of the food chain, we are able to leave the oil intact, including the often missing Phytoceramides. We also include other fat-soluble ingredients, including a standardized amount of Safranal, a carotenoid concentrated from Saffron, the world's most expensive spice. Saffron has been found to improve vision.

Chapter 14

Amino Acids & Polypeptides

Arginine

The cationic amino acid transporter y(+) carries 80% of L-arginine, L-lysine and L- ornithine. Diabetes, chronic kidney failure, and psoriasis are all associated with both L- arginine deficiency and Dry Eye Syndrome.

Chapter 15

Communicators: Hormones & Neurotransmitters

Adrenals & Gonads

Multiple sex hormone issues are linked to Dry Eye Syndrome, although hormone replacement therapies show mixed results, perhaps in part due to synthetic and other non- bio-identical sources, in addition to failure to address underlying causation.

Adrenal Support is a functional formulation we use frequently to restore adrenal function after exhaustion from stress and trauma, or medical steroid treatments.

Autonomic Nervous System

The catecholamine neuro-hormones of stress, like adrenaline (epinephrine), inhibit lacrimal gland secretion, so stress of any kind can contribute to Dry Eye Syndrome.

Stress Release botanical/nutritional capsules and the Infoceutal ESR (Emotional Stress Release) are very effective support for stress management. We also highly recommend a series of ZYTO EVOX sessions to clear current stress patterns followed by clearing inherited epigenetic stress patterns.

Pancreas

One of the first hormonal Dry Eye cases Dr. Sjogren described in 1930 showed insulin resistance. Diabetes is a major cause of Dry Eyes, and correcting glucose metabolism helps reduce dry eye symptoms.

Our two major formulations for this challenge are Glucose Tolerance and Reverse AGE.

Thyroid

Thyroid issues are commonly associated with Dry Eyes. The thyroid receives the highest concentration of Mercury of any body tissue from dental amalgam source.

We formulated Thyroid Support for general Thyroid issues and several remedies to help with Mercury detoxification, especially Glutathione Syntropy and Mercury Detox powder.

Chapter 16

Enzymes: Amplifiers

Antioxidant protection

Antioxidant enzyme levels are reduced in the conjunctiva in Dry Eye Syndrome. Immune function

The immune proteins lysozyme and lactoferrin are reduced in the tears of Dry Eye. Other proteins are often deranged as well.

For the antioxidant factor, we formulated a remedy with the complete intracellular antioxidant system, including antioxidant enzymes. It's called Vitamin C Syntropy.

For immune issues, the main remedy is Immune Modulation.

Chapter 17

Probiotics: Symbionts

Probiotics

Both oral and topical applications of probiotic flora have been reported to help reduce dry eye symptoms.

Staphylococcus aureus

Occasionally, overgrowth of Staphylococcus aureus is present in the tears of people with Dry Eye Syndrome, which is not surprising considering the deficiency of the antibacterial proteins lysozyme and lactoferrin.

Our most popular remedy is our Microbiome because so many people can tell it is really helping when they take it. It is a broad-spectrum probiotic now with 33 species at the time of writing this update.

Before ever considering that you have a deficiency of an antibiotic that never existed in your genetic history (i.e., a fungal toxin analog), beef up your Microbiome. If you have a bacterial imbalance in the mouth, sinuses, eyes, throat, or lungs, open the capsule and take a little powder before you close the capsule and swallow the rest for the gut.

Chapter 18

Fiber

Chitosan-N-acetylcysteine eye drops are being tested for the treatment of Dry Eye Syndrome. For information on oral use of the two detoxifying components Chitosan (fiber) and N-AcetylCystein (sulfur-bearing amino acid), see my book Materia Medica.

Oral fiber intake is crucial for both detoxification and prevention of intoxication from dietary toxins such as heavy metals. Fiber is one of the key missing ingredients in the modern refined and processed food diet.

My three favorite fiber formulas, all of which include a good amount of Chitosan, are:

Binder Complex, for binding and removing the full range of toxins from the gut. Be sure to take extra water with any of these fiber formulations...

Fiber Cleanse is a fabulous balanced fiber for supporting detoxification and peristalsis.

Soothe, formulated to support the relief of constipation.

Chapter 19

Botanical Allies

Artichoke (*Cynara scolymus*) decoction (boiled 10 min.) is used as a moistening eye drop or compress.

Chamomile (*Matricaria chamomilla*) is an anti-inflammatory herb sometimes used as a compress on the eyelids.

Cucumber (*Cucumis spp.*) slices on the eyelids are soothing, moisturizing and anti- inflammatory.

Eyebright (*Euphrasia*) is used topically in the eye as an eyewash to relieve the soreness accompanying dry eye.

Fennel (*Foeniculum*) compresses can help restore moisture to dry eyes.

Mallow (*Mallow sylvestris*) strained infusion (1 tsp/cup as a tea) is used as a soothing, demulcent eyedrop.

Plantain (*Plantago major*) decoction (boiled 15 minutes) is used as a soothing anti- inflammatory eyewash.

Potato (*Solanum tuberosum*) raw slices are placed on the eyelids as an anti-inflammatory. Tea (*Camellia sinensis*) is anti-inflammatory as a compress on the eyelids.

We've formulated lots of angelic Botanical volunteers into our 150+ Functional Formulations, including some specifically for Dry Eye Relief. You can learn more at DryEyeLab.com, as well as our store at RemedyMatch.com. Many people's favorite is Moisturize. You can feel the increase in tear production, and the main side effect of the main botanical ally in the formula is increased longevity!

Chapter 20

Signals: Homeopathy, Sarcodes & Nosodes

Excessive watering of the eyes is sometimes related to dry eye syndrome. This paradox is due to lack of mucin, leading to dry spots which stimulate nerve reflexes to produce more tears in an attempt to rewet the cornea, which contains more nerve endings per square millimeter than any other part of the body. If the excessive tearing, also called epiphora, is due to a blocked tear duct, however, the homeopathic remedy to try is Silicea 6C, taken 4 times a day for up to a week.

Swelling or discomfort around the lacrimal gland, which is superior and temporal to each eye, and lies just posterior the bony orbital rim, can be treated with the Mumps nosode. Other homeopathic remedies for dacryoadenitis include Acontum napellus (monk's hood), Apis mellifica (honey bee), Hepar sulphuris calcareum (impure calcium sulfide, CaS), Iodum (iodine, I), Rhus toxicodendron (poison ivy) and Silicea (silica, SiO2).

Dry eyes may be a contributing factor to the growth of tissue from the conjunctiva onto the cornea. This growth is called a pterygium. Try homeopathic Zinc 6C 3 times a day for 2 weeks, shifting to Ratanhia 6C if no improvement is noticed.

Similisan #1 from Switzerland is available over the counter as a homeopathic complex for dry, red eyes. It contains Belladonna 6X, Euphrasia 6X, and Mercurius sublimatus 6X.

We now supply any individually matching homeopathic remedies, gemmotherapies, botanical tinctures, flower essences, gem elixirs, ORMUS, Oligo Element trace minerals, or other signaling ingredients in a base of Terrain Restore. This replaces traditional carriers which are typically either alcohol or lactose.

Terrain Restore provides many additional healing benefits including healing leaky gut, reducing stress in the kidney tubules, sealing the tight junctions between cells in the vascular endothelium, and sealing the blood/brain and blood/eye barrier. This reduces inflammation throughout the body, and of course, inflammation is a common underlying cause of dry eye issues, as are gut issues. Kidney stress is also strongly related to issues in the front of the eyes.

You can learn more about Terrain Restore at our online store Re medyMatch.com.

We also highly recommend Infoceuticals selected to match your body's healing priorities. We provide free lifetime access to the 10-second online voice scans, which you can do either on your phone or your computer. Click the link at WellnessWhispering.com to set up your free lifetime account.

Chapter 21

Quantum Energy: Color, Light and EMF

Individualized application of Energy Medicine therapies, including the use of photonic, electrical, and magnetic energies to selected points and areas in and around the eyes, can be very helpful in unraveling Dry Eye Syndrome. See my book, Anima Medica, for more details on many of these applications.

Near Infrared

Subjective symptom scores and subjective face scores improved significantly, from 12.3 (SD 5.9) to 8.4 (6.1), and from 7.0 (1.7) to 5.3 (2.0) (both p <0.0001) with Near Infrared treatment for blocked meibomian glands without inflammation. Tear evaporation rates (p = 0.002), fluorescein staining (p = 0.03), rose bengal staining (p = 0.03), BUT (p <0.0001), and meibomian gland orifice obstruction (p <0.0 001) improved significantly with 2 weeks of Near Infrared therapy. (E

Goto, Y Monden, Y Takano, A Mori, S Shimmura, J Shimazaki, and K Tsubota. Treatment of non-inflamed obstructive meibomian gland dysfunction by an infrared warm compression device. Br J Ophthalmol. 2002 December; 86(12): 1403–1407. PMCID: PMC1771385)

My Favorite Therapies:

My favorite approach to healing the eyes is to heal the whole person. Some of the most effective therapies involve energy medicine and are ideal for implementation in the home. That way you can use them every day in the case of Microcurrent and PEMF, or every other day in the case of Infrared soft laser therapy. Skipping a day gives plenty of time for both detoxification and regeneration.

My favorite Microcurrent device is the Denas because it uses biofeedback to send the right signals to balance tissue, whether it is inflamed or degenerative to start with.

My favorite PEMF mat is the Kloud. It applies a full spectrum of sound frequencies all the way up to 20,000 Hz in the form of gently varying magnetic frequencies. Like the BEMER, it restores 40 years of circulation lost to aging by increasing both blood and lymph flow by 30%.

Chapter 22

Acupuncture & Electro-Acupuncture

Therapeutic Acupuncture and Electroacupuncture

In a controlled study, the effectiveness of Electroacupuncture was 79.2%, and of Acupuncture was 56.5%, with the difference showing statistical significance (P<0.05). Both Acupuncture and Electroacupuncture improved eye symptom score, Schirmer I test (SIT), Break-up Time (BUT) of tear film, Corneal Fluorescein Staining (CFS), and Visual Analogue Scale (VAS) values (P<0.001). In particular, Electroacupuncture was more effective at reducing symptoms and improving the Schirmer tear test (both P<0.05).

(Meng-hu Guo, En-cao Cui, Xin-yuan Li, Lei Zong. Diverse needling methods for dry eye syndrome: A randomized controlled study. Journal of Acupuncture and Tuina Science, April 2013, Volume 11, Issue 2, pp 84-88.)

Diagnostic Electroacupuncture

The eye points around the orbital rim include relevant electrodermal measurement points for the Anterior Segment of the eye (Endocrine point 21) located at the lateral orbital margin at the junction of the zygomatic bone with the frontal bone, and the Cornea (Orbit point 11), the Conjunctiva (Orbit point 12) and the Eyelid (Orbit point 13), all located on the inferonasal orbital margin of the Maxillary bone, at approximately 20, 30 and 40 degrees respectively from a vertical line passing through the center of the eye in primary gaze.

The neural loop that regulates the tear reflex is carried by the Trigeminal nerve (CN V) on the sensory side from the cornea and by the Facial nerve (CN VII) on the motor side to the lacrimal gland. The electrodermal measurement point for the Trigeminal nerve is located in the hollow on the superior margin of the zygomatic arch, 1 pouce (thumb width) anterior to the anterior edge of the ear. The point for the Facial nerve (Endocrine point 16a-1) is in the sulcus between the sternal portion and the clavicular portion of the sternocleidomastoid muscle, about 7 fen (about 23 mm, since 1 fen = about 3.33 mm) above the angle of the mandible when the head is in its normal position. This point is only about 5 fen above the measurement point for the Deep Cervical Lymph Nodes (Endocrine point 16a).

Testing these eye and related cranial nerve points can help isolate underlying pathophysiological causes and identify potentially effective remedies by functional response through Medication testing, as discovered in Germany by Dr. Voll in 1953, and as used in select hospitals and clinics in both Germany and Israel. This is also the approach used by some of the royal family in Great Britain and Hawaii.

Chapter 23

Diagnostic Tests

Case History:

A good way to diagnose dry eye is by the history. Patients with dry eye complain of sandy/gritty irritation, burning, or a foreign body sensation that gets worse later in the day. If a patient has these symptoms, they have dry eye until proven otherwise. This is because eye closure at night blocks evaporation, giving the eyes a chance to recover.

Upon eye opening evaporation begins, and symptoms become worse as the day goes on.

There are two main ways that tear film can lose water, increasing tear film osmolarity and causing dry eye:

Decreased tear production

Increased tear evaporation

Tear production decreases with lacrimal gland disease (e.g. Sjögren's syndrome), and anything that decreases corneal sensation:

long-term contact lens wear (hard > soft, extended-wear > daily wear) diabetes

LASIK

PRK (< LASIK)

Herpes zoster

Herpes simplex

Tear evaporation increases with:

Large palpebral apertures, whether anatomical or due to thyroid eye disease meibomian gland dysfunction due to chronic meibomianitis

History: Ask about:

Contact lens wear

Diabetes

Past history of refractive surgery

Past history of herpes infections

Central facial flushing

Look at facial skin for telangiectases. Have the patient look directly ahead at your ipsilateral eye, and measure palpebral fissure width with a millimeter rule. Examine the lid margin, especially the meibomian gland orifices. If you can see them, they are "patent." If you can't see them, but when you press on the lid you see oil come out, they are "stenosed." If you can't see them, and when you press on the lid nothing comes out, they are "closed." The more stenosed and closed meibomian gland orifices, the more meibomian gland dysfunction. Based on palpebral fissure width and assessment of the meibomian gland orifices, you can assess evaporative stress.

Take a fluorescein strip, wet it with some sterile saline, shake off the excess, pull the lower lid down, and paint the strip across the inferior tarsal conjunctiva. Turn the cobalt blue light on, have the patient blink a few times, and then observe the tear film. In early dry eye, the nasal inferior marginal tear strip won't fluoresce. As the tear volume decreases, increasing areas of the tear film won't fluoresce. If the tears are not fluorescing, add a drop or two of sterile saline to the tear film to make the tears fluoresce, improving your view. As the upper lid rises after a blink, the tear film, rather than snapping up with the upper lid, will move more slowly, taking on a more viscous appearance. In drier eyes, debris is visible floating in the tear film. Any of these signs indicates decreased tear production.

With fluorescein in the eye, look at the staining pattern. In mild dry eye, there is no staining. The first place that stains is the exposed nasal conjunctiva, followed by the exposed temporal conjunctiva. The inferior cornea stains last. Even in the late stages of dry eye, the conjunctiva stains more than the cornea. Rose Bengal or lissamine green makes staining more prominent.

Test corneal sensitivity if the history includes risk factors for decreased reflex tearing such as ocular surgery or herpes.

In contrast, meibomianitis patients have symptoms worse on waking because the inflamed eyelids are up against the cornea all night. With meibomian gland dysfunction, the tear film appears more watery. The oil layer, in addition to preventing tear film evaporation, also lowers the surface tension of the tear film, helping to keep it close to the eye. Without the oil layer, tears act more watery and splash out of the eye. (Without the oil layer the Schirmer strip can wet more, giving false negative readings in dry eye.)

Tear film osmolarity in dry eye patients versus normal controls has a sensitivity (positivity in the presence of disease) in the high 90s and a specificity (negativity in the absence of disease) in the high 90s. Measure late in the day.

Specific Risk Factors

Sucrose/folic acid (high dietary ratio over $6 \times 10\text{-}2$ tsp/mcg) increases the risk of low tear film BUT (break-up time) of less than 10 seconds by a factor of 40.

Potassium (dietary intake less than 2500 mg/day) increases the risk of low tear film BUT (<10 seconds) by a factor of 15.

Hair K and/or Na extremely low (K = potassium <8 ppm; Na = sodium <12 ppm for the nape of neck hair) in dry eye syndrome

Tear Na is extremely low in dry eyes. Tear K is extremely low in dry eyes.

Other Tests:

Fatty-Acid Profile of the blood can help to show if there is a need for GLA (e.g. EPO: Evening Primrose Oil) supplementation.

Chapter 24

Energetic Biocommuniation

We now have methods of biocommunication with the body's life force so that in-person office visits are no longer needed to determine the underlying causal stress patterns the body is ready to heal. These methods developed over the past 40 years from the German Diagnostic Electroacupuncture procedures introduced in a previous chapter.

Our first line of testing is now through a simple 10-second voice analysis from an amazing company in London, England, called Nutri-Energetic Systems (NES). Until a few years ago their test required some hardware at the client's location to read the body's biofield. That scanner is still essential for testing young children, animals, and anyone who is non-verbal, such as a client in a coma. If you can count to 10 out loud, though, and you can connect to the internet on your phone or computer, you can now get Bio-energetic Wellness Scan results immediately without any hardware.

Free Online Test (Lifetime Access):

Since you made it this far, you deserve something very, very special:

Go to WellnessWhispering.com and click the button to get a free lifetime account for Voice Scans. A scan takes 10 seconds and you'll have access to the results immediately.

It's one of the energetic tests we use to understand what your body needs to heal the underlying causes of health challenges.

Directions for doing your free voice scan after setting up your free account:

- How to Do a Voice Scan:

  - Log into your account

  - Go to the Scans tab

  - Click the blue button at the upper left that says "BWS Voice Scan" and follow the directions

  - You'll be asked to connect your microphone, which is only necessary the first time you scan, and you'll count from 1 to 10 when prompted...

  - You will get immediate access to your multipage interactive online "**Available to View**" report, and we will be notified and given access to the data, too... You don't need to download the "Complete Report" which is like a whole ebook.

Infoceutical Protocol

You now have access to it free for life. I recommend scanning about monthly and ordering the recommended Infoceuticals. They are drops you put in a little drinking water once a day. If you can drink water, you can do this powerful therapy to turn on your healthy genes, and turn off genes of stress and disease. We work with many people who are very sensitive, so we recommend being gentle as you start each new program. Take only one drop of each Infoceutical on Day 1, and increase by one drop a day until you reach the full dose, which is usually 28 drops a day.

If you experience any increase of symptoms or a return of an old symptom, especially during the first 7 to 10 days of any new healing program, it is likely what we call a healing crisis or cleansing reaction. In that case, take a day or two off the new remedies to give your body a chance to catch up with the elimination of toxins and wastes being released by your cells and tissues.

When you are ready, you can start back where you left off, or even the next lower dosage if your reaction was strong. With a mild cleansing reaction, you can also choose to simply stay at the same dosage level until the symptoms clear, often within a few days.

Functional Formulations:

You can also use your voice scan results to find your Perfect Remedy Matches at RemedyMatch.com, our online store...

Look up each of the Infoceuticals that tests in the Purple range, or at least the five in the Recommendations tab. You'll open the search bar on RemedyMatch.com by clicking the magnifying glass icon in the upper right corner of the page. You can search for part of the Infoceutical name and then click on its image in the search results.

Go to the bottom of the page to select a Functional Formulation that matches your needs from among the Related Products.

Learn More:

You can join our non-profit's free interactive online community to learn more in the free Wellness Whispering course, the free Dry Eye Relief course, and much more!

You can ask questions in the Q&A section, and share with other members... We even offer weekly open office hours through the community so you can meet with us face to face on a video conference.

Your Next Step:

Please complete our online application so we'll have your background information in our clinical database ahead of any video consultation session so we can recommend solutions and program options and answer any questions about your unique health challenges and goals.

The link is:

truly.vip/now

There is no cost or obligation to apply to work with us, and we have programs for every budget.

Join Our Team:

If you feel called to work with us, you can join our team of Affiliates at RegenerateVision.com.

If you want to learn how to help people heal themselves as a coach or practitioner, we can help you get equipped. We can train you and certify you in our methods so you can help us reach and help many more people who are in need and seeking support. The best way to start is to experience our system step by step as outlined above. When you complete your application, you will be letting us know the details of your needs, your interests, your qualifications, and your plans.

We rely on our clients' local eye doctors and other health practitioners to monitor the progress of Accelerated Self Healing™. As we build our network of participating providers who are familiar with and utilize our healing system, we are able to refer our clients to those doctors who are equipped to do more advanced Medicine of the Future.

If you know a great doctor or other healer in your area who would be a perfect fit for us to meet, we would love to have your support in making the introduction. If the relationship is a hit, we make it a win for you as well, so thank you in advance for helping us expand our team – and for being a crucial part of the team!

Chapter 25

Functional Formulations

I started researching and writing this book in 1982, when I became an eye doctor. For 30 years, I printed and bound it for use in our clinic and our research foundations. Then, in 2012, I published it to the rest of the world.

Since then, I have been actively researching and developing over 150 Functional Formulations to better solve the healing needs of our clients and the doctors who use our methods. Now, a dozen years later, it's time to revise this book and add information about those formulations, so you can get direct access.

Dry Eye Relief Program

The Dry Eye Relief Program provides an automatic monthly supply of key remedies to support eye comfort and healthy tear production including:

ACES Eye Drops (1 drop in each eye, AM and PM)

Moisturize capsules (1 per day with food)

WholOmega capsules (4 per day with the heaviest meal)

The cost of these remedies, when purchased separately, is $369.91. When ordered as a monthly autoship package your cost is reduced to $249.97.

You can visit RemedyMatch.com to order the package, or to learn more about each of the Functional Formulations.

If your dry eye issues need additional support, try adding our Moisture Eyes Night Oil.

For deep healing of the root causes of all your health challenges, including dry eye syndrome, go back to the previous chapter and be sure to get on board the Accelerated Self Healing™ process.

Chapter 26

References

Memmert, R., 'Americans fall short of eyecare goals,' 20/20 September 1990, p.44. 'In the News,' Review of Optometry, October 15, 1997, p. 8. (reporting on a study by EagleVision)

Sardi B. Nutrition and the Eyes, Vol. 1. Montclair, California: Health Spectrum Publishers, 1994, p.118-9.

Simmons P.A., et al, 'Toxic effects f opthalmic preservatives on cultured rabbit corneal epithelium,' American Journal of Opthomety & Physiological Optics 65:867-73, 1988.

Simmons P.A., Clough S.R., Teagle R.H., Jaanus S.D., 'Toxic effects of opthlamic preservatives on cultured conrneal epithelium,' American Journal of Optometry & Physiological Optics 65:867-73, 1988.

Gobbels M., Lemp M., 'Artifical tears: preservative's role evaluated,' Opthalmology Times, p.1 and 28, February 15, 1992.

Gobbels M., Spitznas M., 'Corneal epithelial permeability of dry eyes before and after treatment with artifical tears,' Opthalmology 99:873-78m 1992.

Salonen E.M., Tervo T., Beuerman R., 'Toxicity of ingredients in artificial tears and opthlmic drugs in a cell attachment and spreading test,' Journal of Toxicology and Ocular Toxicology 10:157-66, 1991.

Gobbels M.J., Achten C., Spitznas M., 'Effect of topically applied oxymetazoline on tear volume and tear flow in humans,' Graefe's Archive Opthalmology 229:147-49, 1991.

Laflamme M.y., Swieca R., 'A comparative study of two preservative-free tear substitutes in the management of severe dry eye,' Canadian Jouranl of Opthalmology 23:174-76, 1988.

VIVA drops are manufactured by Vision Pharmaceuticals (call 800-325-6789 for a free sample) and are available from Remission Foundation at 800-788-2442, as are individualized non-preserved eye drops in multidose dropper bottles.

Unpreserved eye drops include Refresh, Refresh Plus and Relief from Allergan, BION and Tears Naturale preservative-free from Alcon, Aquasite from CIBA Vision Care and Hypotears preservative free from Iolab.

Sardi B. Nutrition and the Eyes, Vol. 1. Montclair, California: Health Spectrum Publishers, 1994, p.119.

Winfield A.J., Jessiman D., Williams A., Esakowitz L., 'A study of the causes of non- compliance by patients prescribed eyedrops,' British Journal of Opthalmology 74:238-42, 1990.

Burns E., Mulley G.P., 'Practical problems with eye drops among elderly opthalmology outpatients,' Age and Ageing 21:168-70, 1992. Sardi B. Nutrition and the Eyes, Vol. 1. Montclair, California: Health Spectrum Publishers, 1994, p.120.

Smith S.E., 'Eyedrop instillation for reluctant children,' British Journal of Othalmology, 73: 48-81, 1991.

Mansour, A.M., 'Tolerance of topical preparations: cold or warm?' Annals of Opthalmology 23:21-22, 1991.

Sardi B. Nutrition and the Eyes, Vol. 1. Montclair, California: Health Spectrum Publishers, 1994, p.121.

Waltz K.L., 'Contamination of dropper bottles in a glaucoma clinic,' Scientific Poster 141, American Academy of Opthalmology Meeting, October 1990.

Waltz K., Sherwood M.B., 'Ring around the bottle,' release from the American Academy of Opthalmology, October 28, 1990.

Sardi B. Nutrition and the Eyes, Vol. 1. Montclair, California: Health Spectrum Publishers, 1994, p.122.

Sardi B. Nutrition and the Eyes, Vol. 1. Montclair, California: Health Spectrum Publishers, 1994, p.123.

White, W.L., 'Eye drops work better with two minutes of shuteye,' American Acadmey of Opthalmology News Release, October 28, 1990.

Zimmerman T.J., 'Getting a drop on the eye,' Research to Prevent Blindness Science Writers Seminar.

Programs for NeuroFitness Training including these and other eye relaxation techniques are available from RemedyMatch.com.

Tuberville A., et al, 'Punctal occlusion in tear defciency syndrome,' Opthalmology 89:1170-72, 1982.

Willis R.M., et al, 'The treatment of aqueous deficient dry eye with removable punctal plugs,' Opthalmology 94:514-18, 1987.

Tusbota K., 'The effect of wearing spectacles on the humidity of the eye,' Opthalmology 108:92, 1989.

Sardi B. Nutrition and the Eyes, Vol. 1. Montclair, California: Health Spectrum Publishers, 1994, p.125.

Talal N., 'How to recognize and treat Sjogren's Syndrome,' Drug Therapy, June 1984, pp. 80-87.

Leuenberger P.M., 'Cyclosporin, steroids may avert destruction of lacrimal gland,' Opthalmology Times, September 15, 1991, p.35.

Polorny G., et al, 'Primary Sjogrens syndrome from the viewpoint of an internal physician,' International Opthalmology, 15: 401-06, 1991.

Sardi B. Nutrition and the Eyes, Vol. 1. Montclair, California: Health Spectrum Publishers, 1994, p.118.

Khurana A.K., et al, 'Hospital epidemilogy of dry eye,' Indian Journal of Opthalmology 39:55-58, 1991.

Basu P.K., et al, 'The effect of cigarette smoke on the human tear film,' Canadian Journal of Opthalmology 13:22-26, 1978.

Sardi B. Nutrition and the Eyes, Vol. 1. Montclair, California: Health Spectrum Publishers, 1994, p.126.

Frank C., 'Fatty layer of the precorneal film in the office eye syndrome,' Acta Opthalmologica 69: 737-43, 1991.

Bartlett JD. Medications and contact lens wear. In: Silbert JA, ed. Anerior segment complications of contact lens wear. New York: Churchill Livingstone, 1994; 482.

Fraunfelder FT, LaBraico JM, Meyer SM. Adverse ocular reactions possibly associated with isotretinoin. Am J Ophthalmol 1985; 100(4):534-7.

Bergmann MT, Newman BL, Johnson NC Jr. The effect of a diuretic (hydrochlorthiazide) on tear production in humans. Am J Ophthalmol 1985; 99(4):473-5.

Koeffler BH, Lemp MA. The effect of an antihistamine (chlorpheniramine maleate) on tear production in humans. Ann Ophthalmol 1980;12(2):217-9.

Seedor JA, Lamberts D, Bermann RB, Perry HD. Filamentary keratitis associated with diphenhydramine hydrochloride (Benadryl). Am J Ophthalmol 1986; 101(3):376-7.

Fraunfelder FT, Meyer SM. Drug induced ocular side effects and drug interactions, 2nd Ed. Philadelphia: Lea & Febiger, 1982.

Nielsen NV, Ericksen JS. Timolol transitory manifestations of dry eyes in long term treatment. Acta Ophthalmol 1979; 57(3):418-24.

Strempel I. The influence of topical beta blockers on the breakup time. Ophthalmologica 1984; 189(3):110-5.

Van Buskirk EM. Adverse reactions from timolol administration. Ophthalmology 1980; 87(5):447-50.

Almog Y, Monselise M, Amog CH, Barishek YR. The effect of oral treatment with beta blockers on tear secretion. Metab Ped Syst Ophthalmol 1983; 6(3-4):343-5.

Gold D.H., "Systemic Associations of Ocular Disorders," International Opthalmology Clinics, 31:83, 1991.

Silbert JA. A review of therapeutic agents and contact lens wear. Journal of the American Optometric Association, 67(3):165-72

Lane BC. The Tear Film: Nutriture Considerations. Presented at the College of Syntonic Optometry annual conference, 1995.

Tsubota K., Nakamora K., 'Dry eyes and video display terminals,' The New England Journal of Medicine, February 25, 1993, p.584. For more information, see Electromagnetic Pollution Solutions by Dr. Glen Swartwout.

Maury C.P.J., Tornroth T., Teppo A.M., 'Atrophic gastritis in Sjrogrems Syndrome,' Arthritis and Rheumatism, 28:388-94, 1985.

Boyle J., 'The digestive system and Sjogren's syndrome,' Sjogren's Digest, 4:5, 1993.

Cater R.E., 'The clinical importance of hypochlorhydria,' Medical Hypotheses, 39:375- 83, 1992.

Sardi B. Nutrition and the Eyes, Vol. 1. Montclair, California: Health Spectrum Publishers, 1994, p.136.

Testing is available from Great Smokies Medical Lab.

Sherwood L., Gorbach M.D., Goldin B.R., 'Nutrition and the gastrointestinal microflora,' Nutrition Reviews, 50:378-81, 1992.

Sardi B. Nutrition and the Eyes, Vol. 1. Montclair, California: Health Spectrum Publishers, 1994, p.138.

Lane BC. The Tear Film: Nutriture Considerations. Presented at the College of Syntonic Optometry annual conference, 1995.

Roberts H.J., 'Aspartame-associated dry mouth,' Townsend Letter for Doctors, March 1993, p. 201-02.

Tarail J., 'Sjogrens Syndrome: A dry-eyed diary,' American Journal of Nursing, March 1987, pp.324-29.

Khurana A.K., et al, 'Hospital epidemiology of dry eye,' Indian Journal of Opthalmology 39:55-58, 1991

Sardi B. Nutrition and the Eyes, Vol. 1. Montclair, California: Health Spectrum Publishers, 1994, p.138.

Horrobin DF and Campbell AC, 1980. Manthorpe R., et al, 'Primary Sjogrens syndrome treated with Efamol,' Danish Rheumatology Society, June 1983.

Horrobin D.F., Clinical Uses of Essential Fatty Acids, Eden Press, 1982, pp. 129-37.

Schafer D.L., 'Vitamin supplements found to help raise Schirmer value tear volume,' Ocular Surgery News, November 1986

Sardi B. Nutrition and the Eyes, Vol. 1. Montclair, California: Health Spectrum Publishers, 1994, p.129.

Sardi B. Nutrition and the Eyes, Vol. 1. Montclair, California: Health Spectrum Publishers, 1994, p.137.

McLenachan J., 'New aspects of the aetiology of Sjorgrens Syndrome,' Transactions of the Ophthalmological Society, 76:413-26, 1956.

Sardi B. Nutrition and the Eyes, Vol. 1. Montclair, California: Health Spectrum Publishers, 1994, p.130.

Holly F.J., 'Vitamins and polymers in the treatment of ocular surgace disease,' American Academy of Optometry, New Orleans, LA, December 11, 1989.

McLenachan J., 'New aspects of the aetiology of Sjorgrens Syndrome,' Transactions of the Ophthalmological Society, 76:413-26, 1956.

Lane BC. The Tear Film: Nutriture Considerations. Presented at the College of Syntonic Optometry annual conference, 1995.

Lockie A. The Family Guide to Homeopathy; Symptoms and Natural Solutions. New York: Simon & Schuster, 1989; p. 160.

Gold D.H., 'Systemic Associations of Ocular Disorders,' International Opthalmology Clinics, 31:83, 1991.

Horrobin and Campbell, 1980. Lane BC. The Tear Film: Nutriture Considerations. Presented at the College of Syntonic Optometry annual conference, 1995.

Lane BC. The Tear Film: Nutriture Considerations. Presented at the College of Syntonic Optometry annual conference, 1995.

Horrobin D.F., Clinical Uses of Essential Fatty Acids, Eden Press, 1982, pp. 129-37.

Manthorpe R., et al, 'Primary Sjogrens syndrome treated with Efamol,' Danish Rheumatology Society, June 1983

Schafer D.L., 'Vitamin supplements found to help raise Schirmer value tear volume,' Ocular Surgery News, November 1986.

Sardi B. Nutrition and the Eyes, Vol. 1. Montclair, California: Health Spectrum Publishers, 1994, p.135.

Sardi B. Nutrition and the Eyes, Vol. 1. Montclair, California: Health Spectrum Publishers, 1994, p.136-8.

Lane BC. The Tear Film: Nutriture Considerations. Presented at the College of Syntonic Optometry annual conference, 1995.

Horrobin and Campbell, 1980. Sardi B. Nutrition and the Eyes, Vol. 1. Montclair, California: Health Spectrum Publishers, 1994, p. 136.

Paterson C.A., et al, 'Vitamin C levels in human tears,' Archives of Opthalmology 105:376-77, 1987.

Lane BC. The Tear Film: Nutriture Considerations. Presented at the College of Syntonic Optometry annual conference, 1995.

Boyd T.A.S., Campbell F.W., 'Influence of ascorbic acid on the healing of corneal ulcers in man,' British Medical Journal, November 18, 1950, pp.1145-48.

Horrobin D.F., Clinical Uses of Essential Fatty Acids, Eden Press, 1982, pp. 129-37.

Manthorpe R., et al, 'Primary Sjogrens syndrome treated with Efamol,' Danish Rheumatology Society, June 1983

Schafer D.L., 'Vitamin supplements found to help raise Schirmer value tear volume,' Ocular Surgery News, November 1986.

Holly F.J., 'Vitamins and polymers in the treatment of ocular surgace disease,' American Academy of Optometry, New Orleans, LA, December 11, 1989.

Sardi B. Nutrition and the Eyes, Vol. 1. Montclair, California: Health Spectrum Publishers, 1994, p.137.

Lane BC. The Tear Film: Nutriture Considerations. Presented at the College of Syntonic Optometry annual conference, 1995.

Horrobin and Campbell, 1980. Lane BC. The Tear Film: Nutriture Considerations. Presented at the College of Syntonic Optometry annual conference, 1995.

Cotlier, 1983. Lane BC. The Tear Film: Nutriture Considerations. Presented at the College of Syntonic Optometry annual conference, 1995.

Lockie A. The Family Guide to Homeopathy; Symptoms and Natural Solutions. New York: Simon & Schuster, 1989; p. 160.

Lockie A. The Family Guide to Homeopathy; Symptoms and Natural Solutions. New York: Simon & Schuster, 1989; p. 166.

Nosode Therapy in Practice. Baden-Baden, Germany: Biologische Heilmittel Heel GmbH, 1985; p. 63.

Moffat JL. Homeopathic Therapeutics in Ophthalmology. New Delhi, India: B. Jain Publishers, 1982; p. 128.

Lockie A. The Family Guide to Homeopathy; Symptoms and Natural Solutions. New York: Simon & Schuster, 1989; p. 164.

Lane BC. The Tear Film: Nutriture Considerations. Presented at the College of Syntonic Optometry annual conference, 1995.

Lane BC. Fed Proc 1984; 43(March): 1052. Lane BC. Poster at NYAO lecture, 1983.

Gorn RA. 1981 lecture. reported byLane BC. The Tear Film: Nutriture Considerations. Presented at the College of Syntonic Optometry annual conference, 1995.

Available from Monroe Medical Laboratory, Southfield, NY 10975. Levels often improve within 2 months.

Conclusion

The surface of the eye is the most exposed aqueous medium in the human body. It is also the most sensitive nerve center. The tears depend upon the coordination of aqueous, lipid and protein components to maintain the comfort and efficiency of health of the cornea as the first optical medium of our dominant sense, Vision.

This system is exquisitely sensitive to the chemistry of our environment, both internal and external. By supporting all systems of the body to restore balance and harmony in the biological terrain, we give the front of the eye the best opportunity to achieve its design function of accelerated self-healing.

The specific remedies required to achieve this will be different for each individual, and in fact different for the same individual from month to month in the unraveling of the unique individual healing process. Ongoing sources of environmental, dietary, visual and other stress factors will surface as identifiable contributors, and be dealt with in real time as this dynamic healing process unfolds.

This book is intended to help as a resource in that process. Though it can never be complete, if it can facilitate timely identification of one or a few causative or therapeutic factors for you or your challenging patient, then it has fulfilled its primary purpose.

Glossary

AGE: Advanced Glycation Endproducts are the damaging result of excess sugars binding to the body's tissues.

Anti-oxidant: by definition this is an electron donor. The most efficient source of electrons is to ensure we are connected to them from the earth, and are supplying them in abundance in the air and water. This preserves nutritional anti-oxidants for their important co-enzyme functions.

Avascular: lacking a direct blood supply. The interior tissues of the eye, and even the macula lutea in the central retina, in order to be optically clear lack blood vessels once the tissue develops in utero. The remnants of the hyaline artery, active during gestation, cast shadows on the retina, called muscae voluntantes (physiological floaters).

Brunescent: a yellowing of the crystalline lens of the eye.

BEV: see Bio-electronics of Vincent

Bio-Electronics of Vincent (BEV): BEV is an objective means of measuring and calculating energy based on both the electrical (electron) and magnetic (proton) factors in addition to the energetic information factor (photon) via ion content or conductivity (the inverse of resistivity). BEV measurement and analysis can be applied to blood, urine, saliva, water, nutrients, or other substances via measurement of the standard physical parameters: pH, rH2 or O.R.P., and resistivity.

Biokinesiology: Biokinesiology is an advanced method of muscle testing which integrates biocommunication protocols from European electro-dermal testing (see Vegetative Reflex Test and Electroacupuncture According to Voll).

Cataract: a loss of clarity of the crystalline lens of the eye. Clarity of the lens is one of the best known predictors of longevity.

Carrier frequency: A carrier frequency is the frequency or rate at which an oscillating pattern repeats. It acts as the carrier of the information contained in the characteristic pattern of the waveform. The carrier determines the energy content of the individual photons, which transmit the wave. Each specific carrier frequency is like a different AM (amplitude modulation) radio station.

Characteristic waveform: The characteristic waveform is the shape of an electromagnetic oscillation. It is determined by its specific source and represents information content of the electromagnetic oscillation. A characteristic waveform is like the programming on a radio station.

Ciliary Body: the nearest circulation to the lens of the eye, and thus its remote source of nutrition. Like the joints, the lens itself is an avascular tissue.

Crystalline Lens: the lens in the eye that is the densest protein in the body, the most exposed tissue to ionizing radiation, and particularly sensitive to oxidation by free radicals and glycation by sugars (producing AGE), two of the dominant processes of unhealthy aging.

Dowsing: Dowsing is an ancient art of finding water or other substances through amplification of subtle body responses. Dowsers may use wooden or metal dowsing rods, a pendulum, radionic instruments or other convenient amplification devices.

Dry Eye Syndrome: Most often a lack of mucin, the protein which makes the cornea wettable. This is stimulated by Vitamin A, which can be supplied directly in the form of eye drops. More severe cases often involve metal toxicity as well.

Dysbiosis: an imbalance in the normal flora of the body. The body is not a sterile monoculture, but a symbiotic polyculture, right down to the mitochondria, an intracellular bacterium inherited exclusively through the maternal line.

Electroacupuncture According to Voll: EAV is a form of electrodermal remedy testing developed in 1953 by Rheinhold Voll, a German dentist and medical doctor. This system allows the measurement of points and meridians that correspond to specific internal body organs and functions.

Electromagnetic: Electromagnetic field radiation is composed of electrical, magnetic and information components. Electrostatic fields are produced by stationary electrical charges, such as the capacitor in a television set (even when unplugged). Magnetic fields are produced by electrical charges in constant motion, as in a direct current. When electrical charges change their pattern of motion, as in alternating current, electromagnetic radiation is produced. Information is carried in carrier and characteristics waveforms as well as scalar (information only) waves.

Electronic factor: The concentration of electrons in a fluid medium, such as in all biological systems is one of 3 factors, which determine biological energy via the Nernst equation. The other two factors are the magnetic factor and the ion content (electrical conductivity). Because free electrons quickly combine with free protons to produce hydrogen (H_2), their concentration is measured as a function of hydrogen molecules (rH_2).

Fovea Centralis: normally the point of maximum visual clarity, except in night vision, since their are no rod cells in the macular area.

Glaucoma: Wrongly defined as high pressure in the eyes (IOP) even by most physicians, since a high percentage of glaucomatous eyes actually have low pressure. Glaucoma has many patterns related to nutritional deficiencies and toxicities, but is ultimately the result of damage to the optic nerve.

Healing Crisis: this can be a flu-like reaction observed when taking a stimulatory medicine such as homeopathy. It can be based in a cleansing or detoxification reaction,

eliminating stored toxins, or can be a Herxheimer, or die-off process, eliminating bacterial endotoxins or other wastes in the case of dysbiosis.

Hertz: The number of oscillations per second of an electromagnetic field is given the unit Hertz (Hz).

Homeopathy: Homeopathic substances are produced by successive dilution and succussion, resulting in increasing potencies containing increasing electromagnetic carrier frequencies and decreasing chemical concentrations.

Homotoxicology: Homotoxicology is the study of toxins in man. As toxins penetrate further into the system, they may enter more vital organs and tissues. They may also interfere at deeper levels within the cell and ultimately the nucleus. The reversal of this process is marked by a shift in symptoms to more superficial or less vital areas according to anatomy and histology. This detoxification process may also be marked by local metabolism of toxins accompanied inflammatory symptoms, and by increased elimination through mucus membranes, skin, urine or feces.

Homeopathy: the leading form of medicine in the world today in terms of numbers of people treated, and a non-toxic medicine, free of side effects, that works by hormesis, stimulating the body to heal itself by recruiting pathways of response that have been dormant, often due to adaptation to past stresses. Modern science is finally catching up with the field of epigenetics. For over 200 years doctors in this field have watched the non-genetic inheritance of miasms.

Hormesis: The law of dosage effect in pharmacology, also known as the Arndt-Schultz law. Small doses stimulate the body's healing mechanisms. Moderate doses irritate and suppress the ability of those pathways to produce a functional response. Larger doses destroy the same cells.

Ion: A positively or negatively charged particle is an ion. Ions are capable of carrying electrical energy within the body by their movement. The total ion concentration determines the electrical conductivity of a fluid, which is one of 3 factors determining the total energy content according to the Nernst equation. The other two are the electrical and the magnetic factors.

IOP: Intra-Ocular Pressure. High pressure is always an issue, but low or normal pressure does not guarantee health eye tissues and good visual function.

Macula Lutea: the yellow spot in the center of the retina is avascular tissue at the center of which is the Fovea Centralis, normally the point of maximum visual clarity, except in night vision, since their are no rod cells in the macula. The macula has the highest oxygen demand of any tissue in the body, and is energetically linked to the lungs.

Magnetic factor: The concentration of protons, which are positively charged ions, is measured by the magnetic factor (pH). It is one of the 3 basic factors, which determine the amount of biological energy via the Nernst equation. The other factors are the electrical factor and the ion content or electrical conductivity.

Mitochondria: supply 90% of the healthy cell's energy through aerobic metabolism via the electron transport chain, which relies on the B Vitamins as co-factors, and on Oxygen to receive the spent electrons once energy has been extracted for storage and use as ATP.

Muscae Voluntantes: The remnants of the hyaline artery, active during gestation, cast shadows on the retina, as physiological floaters. Toxins in the colon and food reactions can make this shadow darker and more annoying.

Multi-dimensional: Multi-dimensional refers to any process, which has more than just one or two dimensions or key factors. In truth, everything is multi-dimensional. It is only our limited perception, representation or thinking about something that can appear linear (1D) or flat (2D). Space is multi-dimensional (3D). Space-time, which Einstein conceived to be inseparable except by the perception of each individual observer, is 4D. Physicists may now view the universe as 6D, I0D or 26D depending on the context and model proposed.

Nernst Equation: calculates the Energy in a fluid medium, such as biological plasma, in microwatts based on the content of Electrons, protons and Photons.

Ormus: ORMUS is a term used by modern alchemists for an exotic superconductive and superfluid state of the Platinum group of transition minerals with high spin nuclei, also called ORMEs (patented by David Hudson), monoatomic or M-state minerals, and related to the classical Philosopher's Stone as an active universal carrier of consciousness.

Pendulum: A pendulum is a simple device consisting of a suspended weight used to amplify subtle neuromuscular patterns in the arm for the detection of biological responses to subtle electromagnetic energy fields.

Pleiomorphism: Pleiomorphism is the observation of multiple lines of microscopic research, including Enderlein and Naessens, that some endobionts, or symbiotic life forms within the organism, have a reproductive cycle that involves a larger reproductive form that manifests when the symbiotic conditions of the host become imbalanced.

PSC: Posterior Subcapsular Cataract. This is often a fast onset cataract affecting younger people than most other types. It often relates to immune function and typically responds very well to certain remedies including TMG and Cernilton Flower Pollen.

Radiesthesia: Radionics is an approach to detection of biological responses to subtle electromagnetic energy fields using a stick-plate, which is rubbed by the fingertips.

Amplification of subtle physiological changes takes place via noticeable changes in the feel and sound of the stickiness of the stick-plate. Numbers called rates may be used to identify various fields, just as these fields might be identified by names or by numbers such as frequencies, wavelengths, or other characteristics of an electromagnetic oscillation.

Retracing: the tendency to reverse the steps of disease, only much faster in most cases, in the course of the healing process.

Soil Based Organisms (SBO): providing enzyme systems for detoxification, biological transmutation of elements and other functions to assist in altering the course of chronic health issues.

Spectroscopy: A spectroscope measures the intensity of different frequencies of electromagnetic radiation. It is not able to measure the characteristic waveforms of the radiation. The information provided by spectroscopy is therefore like knowing what channels are on the air, but not being able to identify the programming. The most sensitive indicators of the characteristic information in electromagnetic radiation are the physiological responses of biological systems.

Strabismus: an eye that turns in a different direction than its fel-
low eye. Typically eyes turn in with an increase in acidity that causes
increased muscle tension in the extra-ocular muscles, since the Medial
Rectus muscles have the largest cross sectional diameter.

When the metabolism becomes blocked by an even larger accu-
mulation of the toxin, the pH swings to alkaline, and muscle tone
drops below normal, resulting in an outward eye turn. In the course
of restoring healthy function, it is often observed that the outward
tendency (exo) will convert to inward (eso) on its way to restoring
balance. This reversal of the pathway of disease in the healing process
is called the eso-exo swing in this context, and in general is a form of
retracing.

Vegatetative Reflex Test: Formerly called the Vegatest Method,
developed in 1979 by Dr. Helmut Schimmel, this is a method of
electronic monitoring of skin resistance at an acupuncture point.
Homeopathic stimuli are used to determine the patterns of causality
and relief from stress at that time.

Vincent: see Bio-electronics of Vincent

Vitreous Body: the jelly like substance filling the back part of the
eye, behind the lens. This is where most floaters occur. The vitreous is
energetically linked to the large intestine.

Bibliography

Alternative Medicine: The Definitive Guide (Compiled by The Burton Goldberg Group, Future Medicine Publishing, Inc., Puyallup, Washington, 1993).

Balch JF and Balch PA. Prescription for Nutritional Healing. Garden City Park, NY: Avery Publishing Group, 1990.

Berridge EW. Diseases of the Eyes. Jain Publishers, New Delhi, 1984.

Brinker F. Herb Contraindications and Drug Interactions (Eclectic Medical Publications, Sandy, Oregon, 1998).

Burr HS. Blueprint for Immortality: The Electric Patterns of Life (C.W. Daniel Co. Ltd., Saffron Walden, England, 1972).

Chidre D, and Martin H with Beech D. The Heartmath Solution (HarperSanFrancisco, 1999).

Deville M. The Real Trace Element Problem: Their Therapeutic Applications (Centre de Recherches et d'Applications sur les Oligo-Elements).

Dinshah D. Let There Be Light (Dinshah Health Society, Malaga, New Jersey, 1985).

Duke J. Dr. Duke's Phytochemical and Ethnobotanical Databases are online at grin.gov/duke/

Gerber R. Vibrational Medicine: New Choices for Healing Ourselves (Bear & Company, Santa Fe, New Mexico, 1988).

Grossman, M and Swartwout G. Natural Eye Care, An Encyclopedia: Complementary Treatments for Improving and Saving Your Eyes (Keats Publishing, Los Angeles, 1999).

Hahnemann, S. Organon of Medicine (J.P. Tarcher, Inc., Los Angeles, 1982, translated from original written by Samuel Hahnemann 1755—1843.

Hollwich, F. The Influence of Ocular Light Perception on Metabolism in Man and in Animal (Springer Verlag, New York, Heidelberg, Berlin, 1979).

Jackson M and Teague T. The Handbook of Alternatives to Chemical Medicine. (Oakland, California: Teague and Jackson, 1985)

Kappel G. Nutrition and Vision, OEP Foundation, Santa Ana, Calif. 1980. Kavner RS and Dusky L. Total Vision, (AW Visual Library, New York, 1978).

Kenyon, JN. Modern Techniques of Acupuncture: A Scientific Guide to Bioelectronic Regulatory Techniques and Complex Homeopathy (Thorsons Publishing Group, Wellingborough, England, 1985).

Kervran CL. Biological Transmutations (Beekman Publishers, Inc., New York, 1971; originally published in French by L Courrier du Livre, 1966).

Kutsky RJ. Handbook of Vitamins, Minerals and Hormones (Van Nostrand Reinhold Company, New York, 1981).

Lane B. Nutrition and Vision, 273-274, in Bland J, Ed. 1984-85 Yearbook of Nutritional Medicine (New Canaan, Connecticut: Keats, 1985).

Mandel P. Energy Emission Analysis: New Applications of Kirlian Photography for Holistic Health (Synthesis, W Germany)

Mandel P. Practical Compendium of Colorpuncture (Energetik Verlag, Bruchsal, W Germany, 1986).

Manning CA and Vanrenen LJ. Bioenergetic Medicines East and West: Acupuncture and Homeopathy (North Atlantic Books, Berkeley, California 1988).

Moffat JL. Homeopathic Therapeutics in Ophthalmology. Jain Publishers, New Delhi, 1982.

Murphy R. Homeopathic Medical Repertory: A Modern Alphabetic Repertory (Hahnemann Academy of North America, 1993).

Norton AB. Ophthalmic Diseases and Therapeutics. Jain Publishers, New Delhi, 1987.

Ober C, Sinatra ST, and Zucker M. Earthing: The most important health discovery ever? (Basic Health Publications, Inc., Laguna Beach, California, 2010).

Oschman JL. Energy Medicine: The Scientific Basis (Churchill Livingstone, an imprint of Harcourt Publishers Ltd, 2000).

Page LR. Healthy Healing. (Sacramento, California: Spilman Printing, 1990)

Pearson D and Shaw S. Life Extension, A practical scientific approach, (Warner Books, New York, 1983).

Pischinger A. Matrix and Matrix Regulation: Basis for a Holistic Theory in Medicine (Haug International, Brussels, 1991, 1st German edition 1975).

Pizzorno JE and Murray MT. A Textbook of Natural Medicine. Seattle, WA: John Bastyr College Publications, 1987.

Randolph TG and Moss RW. An Alternative Approach to Allergies (Bantam Books, New York, 1980).

Sardi B. Nutrition and the Eyes. (Montclair, California: Health Spectrum Publishers, 1994)

Shils ME, Olson JA and Shike M. Modern Nutrition in Health and Disease, Eighth Edition (Williams & Wilkins, Media, PA, 1994).

Smith CW and Best S. Electromagnetic Man (St. Martin's Press, New York, 1989).

Spitler HR. The Syntonic Principle: Its Relation to Health and Ocular Problems (College of Syntonic Optometry, Eaton, Ohio, 1941).

Stortebecker P. Dental Caries as a Cause of Nervous Disorders (Stortebecker Foundation for Research, Stockholm, Sweden, 1982).

Stortebecker P. Mercury Poisoning from Dental Amalgam - A Hazard to Human Brain (Stortebecker Foundation for Research, Stockholm, Sweden, 1985).

Swartwout GM. Anima Medica: Vis Medicatrix Naturae, 2013.

Swartwout GM. Biofields: The New Physics of Health.

Swartwout GM. Cataract Solutions, 2012.

Swartwout GM. Electromagnetic Pollution Solutions: What You Can Do To Keep Your Home and Workplace Safe, 1991, 2012.

Swartwout GM. Glaucoma Solutions: Prevention and Reversal.

Swartwout GM. Healing Glaucoma, 2012.

Swartwout GM. Macular Degeneration... Macular Regeneration, 2012.

Swartwout GM. Materia Medica: Vis Medicatrix Naturae, 2013.

Swartwout GM. Nous Energy: Healing Power of the Pyramids, 2013.

Swartwout GM. Refreshing Vision: Opening the Windows of the Soul, 2013.

Swartwout GM. The Shire: Glendalf's Guide to Cultivating Your Future Self, 2012.

Swartwout GM. Vision for Living, 1983.

Todd GP. Nutrition, Health & Disease. Norfolk, Virginia: Donning Co., 1985.

Valnet J. The Practice of Aromatherapy: A Classic Compendium of Plant Medicines &Their Healing Properties (Healing Arts Press, Rochester, Vermont, 1980, English translation 1982).

Voll R. 2nd Supplement to the Four Volume Work: Topographical Positions of the Measurement Points of Electroacupuncture According to Voll. EAV Diagnosis of Eye Diseases, 15 New Measurement Points for Portions of the Eye, EAV Therapy for Eye Diseases, 5 New Approaches. Medizinisch Literarische Verlagesellschaft MBH, Uelzen, 1983.

Werbach MR, Murray MT. Botanical Influences on Illness. Tarzana, California: Third Line Press, 1994.

Whang S. Reverse Aging: Scientific Health Methods Easier and More Effective than Diet and Exercise (Siloam Enterprises, Englewood Cliffs, NJ, 1994).

Wurtman RJ, Baum MJ, and Potts JT. The Medical and Biological Effects of Light (The New York Academy of Sciences, New York, 1985).

About the Author

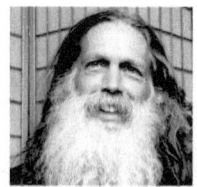

Dr. Glen Swartwout graduated Magna Cum Laude with honors in Environmental Earth Sciences and Chemistry from Dartmouth College, and received his doctorate at the top of his class in Vision Science with honors in Optics as well as Leadership, being inducted into both Beta Sigma Kappa and the Gold Key Honor Societies at the State University of New York in Manhattan, where he trained at the largest outpatient vision clinic in the world. He served as Editor, Vice President, and President of the American Optometric Student Association, serving 4000 international student doctor members. He is the author of over 50 professional papers, books, and software programs. His first professional office was in Tokyo, Japan.

As seen in:

People Magazine (with client, the lovely Carol Merrill of Let's Make a Deal Fame)

USA Today: Dr. Glen Swartwout: Revolutionizing the world of medicine with natural therapies(Truly.VIP/usa)

Science News: Breakthroughs in Reversing Blinding Eye Disease Lead to a New Theory of Everything

Dartmouth Alumni Magazine Cover Story: The Experts: 28 Alumni Share Their Uncommon Knowledge and Tricks of Their Trades: How to Improve Your Vision Naturally (Pictured as The Eye Doctor, next to Daniel Webster, The Statesman)

Also by this author:

Cataract Solutions: Prevention & Reversal Via Accelerated Self-Healing Electromagnetic Pollution Solutions

Healing Glaucoma

Macular Degeneration... Macular Regeneration

Materia Medica: Vis Medicatrix Naturae, Volume 1

Anima Medica: Vis Medicatrix Naturae, Volume 2

Nous Energy: Healing Power of the Pyramids

Refreshing Vision: Opening the Windows of the Soul

The Shire: Cultivating Your Future Self

Dry Eye Relief: Natural Medicine for Accelerated Self-Healing Electromagnetic Pollution Solutions

Biofields: The New Physics of Health

Achievement of Excellence: A Transformational Solution

Additional contributions by the author include:

Alternative Medicine, The Definitive Guide (Vision Chapter)

EPFX SCIO QXCI Quantum Xxroid Eclosion Consciousness Interface (contributor)

IBIS: Interactive BodyMind Information System (contributor)

Natural Eye Care, An Encyclopedia (co-author with Marc Grossman, O.D., L.Ac.)

Transforming Life, Volume 4: 18 Incredible Stories Showing the Strength of the Human Spirit by 18 Inspiring Authors (International Bestselling Series)

TV Series:

A Clinical Theory of Everything

The Five Phases of Disease

The Five Phases of Healing

The Five Tissue Layers

The Five Levels of Regulation

The Five Elements of Spiritual Development

The Hard Question of Consciousness

The Arrow of Time

Find us online:

AcceleratedSelfHealing.com (Our healing system)

AllHeal.org (Non-Profit)

BiofieldAnalysis.com (Our testing)

BiophotonGlass.com (Our bottles)

CataractLab.com

ClinicalPraxis.com (Our methods)

ClinicalTheory.com (Our Theory of Everything)

DryEyeLab.com

EyeHealingCenter.com/Dry-Eye

FunctionalFormulations.com (Our remedies)

HealingGlaucoma.com

IlltoWell.com

GlaucomaLab.com

GlenSwartwout.com (Discover 50+ Website Links)

MacularDegenerationLab.com

MentorshipU.com (Introducing my many mentors)

NutritionalVisionTherapy.com

RegenerateVision.com (Affiliate Funnel)

RemedyMatch.com (Store)

SkepticalReviews.com (Problems with Supplements)

Truly.VIP/now(Application)

WellnessWhispering.com (Get Access to Free Voice Scans)